I0413423

Clean Your Body

Healthy Tips to Do a Body Detox
A Step-by-Step Guide on How to Do a
Safe and Easy Body Detoxification

Sarah Sparrow

PUBLISHED BY:
Sarah Sparrow
Copyright © 2012

Table of Contents

Chapter 1: What is a Body Detox? – All the Information You Need About Detoxification

Body Detox Explained

The whole system of body detoxification involves a series of procedures that include cleansing, resting, and nourishing the body. The entire system leads to natural healing as the body is cleansed from toxic substances and nourished through natural processes.

Dieting and fasting are just some of the common methods used in detox programs. There are also programs that specifically call for the consumption of fruits and vegetables whether in whole or juiced forms.

The utilization of water and herbs are also commonly adapted as these can make the system more effective as a cleansing method. Likewise, foods that contain fats and carbohydrates are avoided as these can lead to poor metabolism.

Different Types of Body Detox

There are 2 main types of body detox, the natural and the artificial type. Both are practiced when aiming to detoxify the major organs of the body.

Natural Body Detox

The liver, kidneys, lungs, digestive system, as well as skin can be detoxified naturally. This will result in a safer method that carries very little side effects, if any.

Fasting

Two of the most popular ways to detoxify naturally is through **water fasting** and **juice fasting**. When these systems are employed, the body can naturally release toxic wastes (chemicals, heavy metals, etc.) by sweating and urinating. Moreover, solid waste matter can be eliminated from the body through the feces.

Water, fruits and vegetables are commonly used in natural body detox methods. Garlic, onion, ginger, as well as plums and peaches can break down the formation of mucous in the lungs so as to detoxify this organ. This promotes proper circulation of oxygen so that it can flow through the entire system through the blood stream.

As the colon is also one of the most contaminated organs of the body, it is also important that this part is detoxified and cleansed regularly. In order to do this naturally, one can simply increase the intake of high fiber fruits and vegetables like spinach (and other leafy veggies), apples, and oranges. These types of produce promote regular bowel movement so that harmful chemicals are not trapped along the linings of the intestines.

Although regular detoxification of the internal organs is essential in keeping a well functioning system, detoxifying the body's largest external organ, the skin, is also very important. Aside from increasing the intake of water so that the body can flush out toxins from the system more efficiently, you can also make use of other methods of detox.

Dry Skin Brushing

Dry skin brushing is a natural means of stimulating the skin so that the pores can open up and release toxic wastes efficiently. This is done by passing the gentle strokes of a brush on the arms and the legs until it reaches the chest area. It is also recommended that this is done before taking a bath so that dead skin cells and other toxic substances in the blood stream can be released through the skin as one cleanses the body.

Cleansing Bath

Going on a **cleansing bath** is yet another way to detoxify the skin. In this method, hydrogen peroxide, Epsom salt and baking soda are mixed together in the bath tub. The combination of these ingredients with hot water act as detox agent as the salt draws out the toxins inside the body to be released out into the water. The baking soda and hydrogen peroxide serve as cleansing and neutralizing agents in this mixture.

Artificial Body Detox

Detox Pills

Taking medication or **detox pills** is also commonly employed in detox programs. However, if the pills contain synthetic ingredients, these can leave harmful chemicals in the body. And if that's the case, the method may bring more harm than good to the body. You see, a detox program aims to reduce toxic substances from the system, and not add more pollutants to the body.

Enema and Colonic Irrigation

Enema and **Colonic irrigation** is also practiced when one chooses to seek medical assistance in cleansing the digestive system. In these methods, water is introduced into the colon through an instrument. The pressure used in the program can then force out the hardened materials that have been trapped in the intestines.

In some methods, herbs and other medicinal substances are mixed with the water before its introduction to the body. Or prescribed medications like laxatives and purgatives may also be used in order to make the system more effective.

How to Detox the Body

There are many ways of detoxifying the body. Going on a **juice diet** is one of the most popular forms of natural body detox as it simply involves the consumption of fruits and vegetable juices. For the duration of the program, all other beverages (coffee, tea, processed juice) are avoided and all forms of solid food are eliminated too. This is a convenient way of cleansing the body as it can still provide for the basic nutrition that's needed by the system.

Water Fasting

Water fasting is yet another method of body detox, and it has been around since time immemorial. In this type of program, only purified water is consumed in order to flush out harmful substances from the body. While it is deemed to be effective and safe in cleansing the system, it should only be adapted for a limited period of time as the body is cut off from getting nutrition from other food sources.

Exercising

Although not intended as a stand-alone method for detox, **exercising** is a natural way of assisting the program. It stimulates the vital organs to work properly, and also releases toxic elements that are trapped inside the body through the skin (by sweating). However, when this method is adapted with other forms of cleansing, it may be necessary to only take on mild forms of exercises in order to preserve the body's energy while undergoing the program.

Dry Skin Brushing

Dry skin brushing is another detox method that can be regularly used as a maintenance for body cleansing. It simply involves the use of a special type of brush that is rubbed on the skin in order to remove dead skin cells and promote efficient functioning of the sweat glands. It is a very simple method that can be carried out without much fuss.

Herbs

The use of **herbs** is also popular among practitioners of body detox programs. This can be taken in as raw by including it in juice diet recipes. There are also supplements that use processed herbs and other natural ingredients. And these can be taken in specified doses depending on one's needs.

Detox Body Wrap

A detox body wrap is typically held in a spa as it needs to follow a complex procedure in order to be truly efficient. The procedure starts with exfoliation so as to open up the pores on the skin. This is done by scrubbing or brushing as the gentle strokes from the friction can unclog the pores and make the skin more conducive to releasing toxins. Once the body is clean and exfoliation is completed, the actual treatment procedure can begin. A mixture of ingredients that can contain seaweed extracts, algae, mud, and other natural ingredients is slathered onto the body to form a body mask. This is then allowed to stay on the body for about 20 minutes or so.

The procedure is carried out by a massage therapist as the body is rubbed down during the process. This gives a stimulating effect so that the internal organs of the body can release toxic waste materials through the skin.

When time is up, the body mask is removed and washed off from the body. And as soon as the body is dried off, a special type of lotion is applied so as to keep the skin moisturized and hydrated.

Ion Detox Bath

When one goes through an ion detox bath, the feet are immersed in a solution of warm water. A special gadget called an ion generator is used and this triggers the production of both positive and negative ions.

The system works by drawing toxic elements from the body through the soles of the feet. This is done as the positive and negative ions attach themselves to oppositely charged toxins that are trapped inside the body. Working as magnets, said toxic substances are pulled out of the body through the skin's pores.

While there are numerous claims as to the effectiveness of the method, the actual effects of the system remain to be questionable as there are no sufficient evidences that can support it. In fact, detractors of the procedure attribute the program's effectiveness to placebo effect wherein the power of the mind can bring about certain positive results. Nevertheless, this type of procedure has been known to alleviate symptoms of rheumatism and arthritis. And there are even those who claim that it can regulate blood pressure and treat certain forms of bodily pain (e.g. headaches, migraines, cramps, etc.).

Processes Involved in Body Detox

One's mental and physical well-being is involved when a person undergoes a body detox. Lifestyle changes are also sometimes called for, as there are certain practices that can be damaging to the health. Habits such as drinking and smoking need to be avoided while going through a detox, and a healthy diet needs to be adapted too.

As the body goes through an intensive processing of releasing toxic substances from the system, you can expect to experience certain uncomfortable side effects. Skin eruptions, stomach upsets as well as headaches and a general feeling of weakness are commonly experienced by those who engage in this program.

As much as there are unpleasant symptoms, however, these are only temporary and short-lived. Note that the body is not really sick but is merely cleaning itself, so you can expect to feel better after the method is successfully completed.

What to Expect When You Do a Body Detox

Because of genetics and lifestyle, different people will have varying reactions to detox methods. However, a feeling of weakness and irritability is generally experienced by many as the body adjusts to the changes in food intake and general routines.

Aside from the physical manifestation of tiredness and lack of energy, one may also observe unpleasant reactions of the body to the cleansing process. There could be an increase in the frequency of bowel movement and urination, and these can be very smelly too. In fact, even the color of the feces and urine may be unusually dark.

A more profuse sweating can also be expected as this is one of the body's natural ways of releasing toxins from the system. Women may even have longer menstruation periods because of the large amount of toxic elements that flow through the blood. However, aside from being less painful than the usual soreness that can be attributed to the condition, one's regular flow can also be expected when the detox program is through.

How to Prepare Yourself Before a Body Detox

No matter what type of detoxification method you choose to adapt, the first thing that you should focus on is your diet. You should abstain from eating solid food a few days before the program as this can leave some hard residue on your intestinal tract. Furthermore, undigested food materials will affect the efficiency of the detox procedure.

At this point, it is also important to give up certain unhealthy habits like drinking and smoking. These will pollute the system further and make it harder for toxic wastes to be eliminated out of the body. Likewise, it would also help if sources of caffeine (coffee, tea), sugar (soda, commercial juices), and preservatives (canned and frozen food) are avoided as these will only aggravate one's level of toxicity.

What You Can Eat After a Body Detox

It is of utmost importance that there is a gradual transition from liquid to solid food so as not to cause any chemical imbalance inside the body. A sudden change in the diet can also cause stomach problems as the system is not yet ready to the new form of food that you introduce to the system.

You therefore need to start with soft diets of soups, broths and juices after an intensive detox procedure. And as the day progresses, you can begin to consume whole forms of fruits and vegetables as well as brown rice.

Other nutritious and safe types of food that you can eat after a detox are yogurt and gelatin. These are both soft and stomach-friendly, and they are delicious as well.

How Many Times in a Week Should You Do a Body Detox?

The frequency of body detox differs from person to person as it will depend on the toxicity level as well as the individual's general lifestyle. The more toxic wastes that the body has, the greater is the need for detoxification.

One's regular diet and habits should also be taken into consideration as exposing yourself to fatty, greasy and food sources that are full of preservatives can pollute the body internally. So if your goal is to cleanse the system, you can adapt a program that runs for about 3 to 7 days a few times in a year. But if your goal is to lose weight, you can detoxify the body regularly about once a week.

Side-Effects of Undergoing a Body Detox

While headaches, weakness, and even breakouts may be experienced while doing a detoxification procedure, these will all go away once the body has adjusted to the method. Diarrhea, nausea, bad breath and body odor can also be expected as these are all forms of toxic waste elimination. However, these side effects of natural body detox only last a few days, unlike the many harmful side effects of prescription drugs that can even lead to long term repercussions.

Moreover, one can reap the rewards of the system once the whole process is completed, and high energy as well as a clearer mind can be achieved. And as the body's immune system is strengthened by the program, you will also be less prone to illnesses.

Will You Feel Weak After Doing a Body Detox?

A person will generally feel weak while doing a body detox as one's usual consumption of energy-giving food becomes limited. The method of cleansing can also have an energy-depleting effect as the body attempts to release all trapped toxic substances from the system. Unlike traditional medications, however, most detox methods use natural ingredients. Therefore, you are not exposed to the harmful side effects that can be attributed to the use of chemicals and unnatural substances.

After completing a body detox procedure, you will immediately feel its positive effects as your energy level starts to increase. Any sluggish feeling will be gone, and you will feel light and relaxed as well. Even your sleeping patterns will improve as the body is now at a more peaceful state.

There are also physical manifestations of a clean system. Aside from losing some of those extra pounds, your skin and overall complexion will also improve. And mentally, you will be more alert and analytical.

Detoxifying Your Body From Toxin Build-Up

Even if the body is free from diseases, an occasional cleansing method is needed to keep it strong and healthy. Everyone is constantly exposed to harmful chemicals in the environment and even in the food we eat, and this puts the body at risk of developing an illness.

Improper eating habits also increases the body's exposure to sickness as food groups that are filled with preservatives and fatty components can clog up the arteries and slow down the body's metabolism too. And if one has the habit of drinking, smoking, and taking drugs, the major organs of the body (e.g. liver and kidneys) are specifically affected.

That's why the body has its own cleansing mechanism that releases toxic substances from the system. However, while regular bowel movement is very helpful in the process of detoxification, it may not be able to handle the high amounts of harmful substances that are present inside the body.

Another way to naturally detoxify the system is through regular exercise as this stimulates the vital organs to function properly. The activity doesn't even have to be too strenuous as even walking, jogging, and climbing the stairs can promote the release of toxic materials through sweating.

And if you want to adapt a system that involves dieting, you can go on a juice fast and eliminate solid foods from your diet for a certain period of time. During the process, the body can get rid of toxins without eliminating the body's source of vitamins and minerals. The method is gentle and less demanding than a water fast, but the consumption of water is also included in the program. This will support the system in efficiently flushing out waste matter from the body.

Can You Still Take Your Prescription Medicines While Doing a Body Detox?

In general, it is not advisable to combine prescription medicines with a detox program. The medicines may affect the efficiency of the procedure, or add more harmful chemicals to the system. Likewise, an intensive detox method may also interfere with the effects of prescription drugs. This can either render the medicines ineffective, or it may even result in a life-threatening side effects.

The best way to conduct a detox procedure is to carry it out without taking in any artificial substances. And in order to ensure one's safety, a physician should first be consulted before undergoing the program. This way, you will know if the detox method is safe for you, and if it's advisable to stop taking medications temporarily.

Do Body Cleansing Programs Really Work?

Detox programs work differently for different people as the body's composition and genetics also vary. Moreover, there are cleansing programs that are proven safe and there are also those that are quite risky.

While colon cleanses are very common today, there are certain types that can be considered harmful. As the system aims to clean out the digestive tract from hardened feces and other toxic matters, the good bacteria that are necessary for proper functioning and digestion are also eliminated. And this puts the body at risk as it becomes more prone to ailments on the stomach area.

The use of laxatives as a colon cleanser or as a weight loss solution should also be approached with caution. Aside from being physically addictive, the ingredients used in this type of medication can be very harsh on the stomach lining and digestive tract.

Kidney and liver cleanses that make use of medicines are also equally risky as the drugs may make use of chemical substances. Unnatural ingredients carry many harmful side effects, and these may bring more harm than good to the body.

If you want a safe way to detoxify the body naturally, you can try out juice diet programs that call for the consumption of fruit and vegetable extracts. As these ingredients are natural, they are safe for the body and highly nutritious as well. By simply increasing one's fiber intake, the body can be efficiently cleansed out of toxic materials. And this is done in a slow and safe manner so as not to strain the system and cause an imbalance to the body's nutritional sources.

You can also go on a water fast. But although the method may seem gentle and safe, it is actually very intense and demanding. While it has been proven effective as a cleansing solution for many generations, it is not as nutritious as juice fasting. The mineral content of water is quite low, and the body will naturally feel weak when the system is carried on for an extended period of time.

Chapter 2: Top Health Benefits of a Body Detox

Why Body Detox is Important to Health

Because of the presence of toxins in the environment and the food we eat, it becomes of utmost necessity to detoxify the body regularly. Not doing so will render the vital organs of the body to function improperly and harmful substances will not be eliminated from the system efficiently. If this happens, the body becomes exposed to different types of diseases as the immune system becomes weak and prone to infections.

By conducting a body detox program, toxic substances can be released from the body systematically. And as this is done naturally, the method can be considered safe and gentle.

Benefits of a Body Detox

One of the main benefits of keeping the body clean and detoxified is that one's immune system is strengthened. This makes it more resistant to germs and even killer diseases.

Regular colon cleansing will also minimize the risk of developing colon cancer as well as other stomach ailments (ulcer, gas, etc.) as the digestive system is kept clean and free of harmful waste products. The method also promotes proper digestion which is beneficial to the body as vitamins and nutrients from the food we eat are more readily absorbed by the system.

Sufferers of diabetes can even benefit from certain types of detox programs as the system is also known to be effective in regulating blood sugar levels. However, as diabetes is a serious problem, detoxification should be done under a doctor's supervision.

The process of body detox can also be helpful to those people with unhealthy habits like drinking and smoking. As these practices pollute the body and slow down its metabolic state, it can hinder the organs from functioning properly. An efficient body detox can effectively eliminate the nicotine substances in the system and even alcohol residue can be flushed out of the body.

An unpolluted system results in an unlimited number of benefits as it can also make the body energetic and full of life. In fact, the method even promotes proper circulation of oxygen which is beneficial to the entire body. Aside from having a clear mind, a clean system also treats sleeping problems.

Do Body Detox Programs Have the Same Benefits as Fasting?

Fasting is a form of detox, and this can be adapted in many different ways. The most intense form of this kind of detox is **water fasting** wherein only water is consumed for the duration of the program. As this method can prove to be too demanding, bed rest is often advised and vigorous activities are temporarily eliminated from one's routine.

A less demanding method of fasting is one that involves the consumption of fruit and vegetable juices. When one takes on juice fasting, solid foods are removed from the diet. This method is not as risky as water fasting, as the body is still supplied with vitamins and minerals.

Both forms of fasting are effective as detox methods as they can both eliminate bodily toxins. However, juice fasting is now considered to be safer and more effective as it proves to be less challenging for the body. And as the digestion process is bypassed by the system, this allows the nutrients from the fruits and vegetables to be readily absorbed by the body.

Allowing the body to rest from digesting hard and fatty foods can effectively clean the system from harmful substances. This then results in well-functioning organs that will benefit the whole body in general.

Chapter 3: Safe and Natural Methods of Detoxification

Natural Home Remedy for Body Detox

Body detox doesn't need to be elaborate and expensive in order to work. You can perform a detoxification program right in the comfort of your own home, using ingredients and methods that are readily available.

Cabbage Soup Detox

A cabbage soup diet needs to be carried out for 7 days in order to serve as a detox method. Basically, you need to add other ingredients to the cabbage, like onions, tomatoes, green pepper, mushrooms, and celery. All these components are helpful in effectively getting rid of toxins inside the body, and the soup will generally taste good too.

In this type of cleansing diet, you can consume as much of the soup as you want to in a day. However, it should be the only food that you consume during the entire 7 days of carrying out the program. An increase of intake in water is also advised, as this will assist the body in flushing out waste materials efficiently through the different organs of the body.

Aside from being an easy-to-prepare home remedy for body detox, the cabbage soup diet can also be performed when getting ready for a weight loss program. As meat products are removed from one's daily regimen, the body is still supplied with essential vitamins and minerals derived from the consumption of vegetables.

Juicing

Juicing is now known as the one of the easiest ways to carry out a body detox at home. The method is safe as you are only using fresh fruits and vegetables in the juice recipes.

You can literally use any type of produce available in the kitchen as long as you can tolerate the taste. You have the option of juicing your favorite fruits, or your favorite vegetables, or combining both for a really nutritious drink.

Fruits and vegetables generally carry fiber, and this is essential in cleansing programs. Just look around your kitchen, and throw into your juicer or blender any type of ingredient that you choose. The most beneficial fruits and vegetables for a detox program include apples, berries, carrots, broccoli, spinach, and other green leafy veggies.

Water

The importance of water in a detox program can't be stressed enough, as this enables the system to effectively flush out impurities, heavy metals, and toxic elements out of the system.

If you have been drinking alcohol, and want to flush out the alcoholic residue from your body immediately, then drinking water is the best way to accomplish this goal. By simply drinking a glass of water every hour for 8 hours straight, most of the alcoholic substances inside your body will be released from your system. This also works for flushing out caffeine when one has been taking in too much coffee or tea.

Fruit Fast

This home remedy is different from the typical juice fasting method as it only involves one type of fruit to make the system work. According to some scientific studies, consuming only one type of fruit for 3 days straight can work in purging out fat, preservatives, and other unhealthy materials that are trapped inside the body.

Apples are the most recommended fruit for this home remedy detox method, and they can be consumed whole or in juice form. The method also involves consuming at least 8 glasses of water each day.

Fruit and Vegetable Dietary Strategy

This type of home remedy should be carried on for 7 days as it involves a very systematic approach. Basically, the program aims to increase one's fiber intake as this will help in effectively absorbing toxins inside the body so that these can be eliminated from the system efficiently.

You can use a wide variety of fruits and veggies for this detox diet as most produce are naturally high in fiber. Avocados, apples, grapes, broccoli, carrots, eggplants and other leafy greens are just some of the ingredients that you can use for this plan.

On day 1, you are to consume 1 pound of fruits and veggies either in raw or steamed form. And on day 2, you are to increase the amount of intake to 2 pounds. You will increase your consumption of fruits and vegetables by 1 pound each day until you complete the 7 day period. Again, water is included in this program as the body needs it to properly eliminate harmful materials from the system.

By the 8th day, the body will start releasing high volumes of waste products from the body. And you will notice this by the bulk of stool released through bowel movement. As you have been eating a wide variety of fruits and vegetables for the entire 7 days, your stool may carry weird colors. And as a sign of toxic release, they can also have some really bad odor.

Fluid Therapy

Not all detox programs call for dieting and limited intake of food. When you adapt a simple fluid therapy, it simply means taking in high amounts of liquids (especially water) all throughout the day. This is especially important with every meal as it helps in the digestion process.

When going through this method, however, you need to limit your intake of caffeinated products like coffee and tea. You see, caffeine is not included in many detox programs because it can hinder the body from releasing toxic substances efficiently. Moreover, liquid products that are high in sugar should also be avoided as it will be counter-productive to the cleansing system. Note that one of the goals of a detox program is to get rid of harmful substances in the system, and that includes sugar and caffeine.

Simple Fasting

There's no question about it that you can carry out a simple type of fasting right at home if you want to. When adapting this method, you will need to eliminate the consumption of meat and other types of food that are loaded with saturated fats, sodium, and sugar.

You can opt to go on a water fast or a juice fast. This can be held for just a day or for an extended period of time (7 days or so).

Fruit and Veggie Detox Plan

When you choose to adapt this type of home remedy, you should avoid eating processed food and other sources of artificial ingredients. Carbonated drinks as well as coffee and tea should also be avoided because of its caffeine content. As you are aiming to fully detoxify your body from toxic elements, drinking and smoking should also be stopped.

This detox plan runs for a duration of 10 days. On the first 2 days, you are to eat only one kind of fruit. Apple is a popular choice as it is considered to be a general cleanser because of its high fiber content (and it's nutritious too!).

If you are particularly aiming to detox your digestive system, then mango and papaya are more recommendable as these are good for the stomach. These fruits are also high in fiber which can help in absorbing toxins from the walls of the intestines before releasing these through bowel movement.

If you are after blood purification, then you can eat grapes for 2 straight days. And if you are acidic, cherries will be more suitable for you as this can neutralize the acids in your stomach during detoxification. You can also eat watermelon for the first 2 days if you are after cleansing the kidneys.

From day 3 to day 10, you are to eat only vegetable products. Green leafy veggies are especially recommended as these are loaded with nutrients and fiber as well. You can consume a wide variety of food on the last 8 days as fruits, nuts, seeds, and grains (brown rice) are also allowed. In fact, you can even eat small amounts of yogurt and cheese. Only meat and milk are strictly prohibited during this time when one is undertaking this detox program.

On the 11th day, you can go back to your normal diet. Just make sure to reintroduce solid food and meat products gradually as your body is still recuperating from the cleansing method. And sudden introduction of food to the system can cause shock, trauma, and stomach upsets.

Edgar Cayce's 3-Day Apple Diet

This is by far one of the easiest home remedies that you can adapt if you want to detoxify your system. You only need a supply of delicious apples to carry out this program.

As the title suggest, you will only be consuming apples during the 3-day cleansing program. So be ready to eat around 5 to 6 apples per day. And at the end of the 3rd day period, you are to take 2 ounces of olive oil (about 2 to 3 teaspoons). The olive oil will initiate the process of detox by releasing toxins through the colon and supplying the body with essential nutrients as well.

During this 3-day program, you will also be required to drink plenty of water (8 glasses or more) as water helps in flushing out harmful substances from the body. And it is also strongly advised that you take a lot of rest as the body may feel weak because of the limited supply of food for 3 days.

Grape Detox Plan

Grape is one also one of the popular ingredients for detox recipes, but it can actually be taken in as it is. You can eat grapes in whole form or juice form, whichever way you enjoy the most.

Grapes are rich in potassium, it therefore aids in keeping the blood and kidneys healthy. Moreover, this element is also good for the heart, so it can regulate proper heartbeat as well.

The high fiber content in grapes also aids in detoxifying the system. When this type of home remedy is adapted often, practitioners will have regular bowel movement.

Asparagus Cleansing Diet

Regular intake of asparagus will naturally cleanse the body of toxic elements. This type of vegetable contains high levels of amino acids, and this will give a diuretic effect to the system. You will therefore urinate often, and release waste materials through the urine. Asparagus is also loaded with fiber, and this promotes regular bowel movement.
If you always have a supply of asparagus in your kitchen, you can add this to your cooking recipes so as to benefit from its cleansing properties. You can also blanch it to serve as a side dish, or include it in your juice recipes.

Pure Cranberry Juice Detox Program

If you love cranberries, then you can use this as a detox home remedy when you are feeling sluggish or out of sync. This type of fruit can lower uric acid, toxins, and purines that are present in the kidneys, prostate gland and bladder. It is therefore the perfect detoxifier for some of the major organs of the body.

Dandelion Cleansing Tea

Dandelion leaves make for a delicious tea, and they also serve as natural blood cleansers. Because of its detox properties, it also functions as a laxative to help ease constipation problems.

Licorice Root Home Remedy

You will benefit from the cleansing effects of licorice root when you use it as an ingredient in your dishes. It can also be added to juice diet recipes so that you can take it fresh and raw.

This root crop has detoxifying effects on the liver, lungs, and kidneys. Aside from stimulating these organs to release waste materials, it also promotes healing.

Green Leafy Vegetables Diet

As a source of roughage, green leafy vegetables can be considered as potent detox agents. Lettuce, cabbage, kale, spinach, and collards are just some of the veggies that fall under this category. These are commonly found in the kitchen, so it's easy to prepare meals with them or blend them into interesting juice recipes.

The fiber contents in leafy greens make them suitable for digestive tract detoxification. As hardened feces may have stuck to the intestinal walls, consumption of these high-fiber produce will enable the system to loosen up the hardened fecal matter so that these can be flushed out from the body through defecation.

Good Sources of Fiber for Body Detox

The body's needed fiber can be generally sourced from plant life. There are 2 major types, the water-soluble fiber and the water insoluble fiber.

Water-soluble fiber assists in the proper circulation of blood, and the lipid component contained therein helps prevent cholesterol and fat build-up. Some examples of this type of fiber include fresh fruits and veggies, seeds, and soybeans.

Water-insoluble fiber, on the other hand, generally works for the digestive system. As it aids in proper digestion, constipation and irregular bowel movement can be avoided. Regular consumption of this type of fiber can also reduce the risk of developing colon cancer as the intestines are kept clean and toxin-free. Whole wheat grains and breads, vegetables, and fruit skins contain this type of fiber.

Fruits

The berry family (strawberries, cranberries, blueberries, raspberries, blackberries) can be regarded as one of the best sources of fiber. Likewise, apples and pears are also commonly used in detox programs because of their cleansing properties. With both types of fruits, however, much of the fiber contents are on the skin. So it would be much better to consume them without peeling off the skin.

Apples, in particular, are said to be capable of absorbing metals and other types of food additives that have penetrated the body. These can then be released through sweating, urinating, and defecating.

Beets

This type of vegetable is a good source of fiber, and it contains iron, zinc, magnesium and calcium as well. Beets are good for the liver, gall bladder, and digestive system as it can break down the toxic elements in these organs. There will be a more efficient removal of toxins when these are no longer clinging to the system.

Seaweeds

Seaweeds are particularly helpful to the digestive tract. They act like a sponge that absorbs toxic elements in the colon so that these can be released through the stools. Because it also acts as roughage, one will not experience irritable bowel movement.

Dandelion leaves

The fiber content in dandelion leaves enables proper cleansing of the digestive tract. Moreover, it also supports the liver by supporting its filtering system. Dandelion leaves are best consumed as tea as it can also provide a soothing feeling to the detox practitioner.

Broccoli

Known as a detox vegetable, you can use broccoli for a wide variety of dishes. Its pleasant taste also makes it a suitable ingredient for juice diet recipes. It contains high levels of fiber, so it promotes regular bowel movement too.

Flaxseed

Flaxseed works as a detox agent as it is capable of binding toxins and then flushing them out of the body. This is particularly helpful in maintaining a healthy digestive system as even stubborn metals and chemicals that have stuck to the intestinal walls can be loosened and eliminated completely.

Natural Ways to Detox the Body

As the body is equipped with an internal mechanism that can promote self-healing, one only needs to stimulate its natural defenses to activate the process. By following certain rules and performing certain tasks, the body can naturally detoxify the system and get rid of harmful elements that are trapped inside the body.

Eat High-Fiber Food Sources

By eating fruits and vegetables that are high in fiber, the body will be able to eliminate waste products through regular bowel movement. Some of the best ingredients for a detox program include beets, cabbages, artichokes, broccoli, and seaweeds among others. As much as possible, you should only consume organic produce so as to avoid pesticides that may still be present in the crops.

Drink Herbal Teas

Natural teas have the capacity to cleanse and protect the vital organs of the body. Green tea, Burdock root tea, and Dandelion tea are just some of the drinks that can detoxify your body while providing for refreshing and soothing effects too.

Take Vitamin C

Aside from eating fruits and veggies that are high in vitamin C, you can also take supplements to help in the detox process. This vitamin stimulates the production of glutathione which can assist in driving toxins out of the system.

Drink Plenty of Water

8 glasses of water is recommended daily. However, if you want to truly detoxify your body, you can consume more than 8 glasses so as to efficiently wash out harmful chemicals from the system.

Practice Deep Breathing

When you get into the habit of breathing deeply, there will be proper circulation of oxygen through the entire system. This will help clean the blood and promote proper functioning of all the major organs of the body.

Avoid Stress

Stress releases adrenalin which is actually harmful for the body. You should therefore try to avoid stressful situations while undergoing a detox program, and adapt a positive mental attitude too.

Sweat It Out in a Sauna

Toxins are released through the lymph and skin when one sweats profusely. However, you should also make sure that you are adequately hydrated by drinking plenty of water so as not to experience shock and dehydration.

Pamper Yourself with Foot Spa

Foot spas will provide you with a soothing feeling and it's an effective way to detox the body too. By massaging and soaking the feet in warm water, toxic elements can be eliminated from the body through the pores on the skin.

Go on a Juice Diet

By using natural ingredients (fruits and veggies) that are present in your kitchen, you can create a lot of juice recipes that can cleanse your body from the inside out. Some of the popular ingredients for juice diet recipes include apples, oranges, pineapple, carrots, spinach, lettuce, and ginger.

Exercise Regularly

By performing certain exercises (even simple routines), the body's organs can be stimulated to release toxic substances. Poisonous elements can then be released through the skin.

Chapter 4: Best Diet Detox Plan – Super Food and Beverage to Clean You Up

What Are Some of the Best Food to Eat to Detox Your Body?

Water

As the body is comprised of a large amount of water, it is also one of its most needed elements. Aside from keeping the body hydrated, it works as a flushing agent in getting rid of harmful substances from the system.

Fruits

Fruits have always been known to carry high amounts of vitamins and minerals that are beneficial to the body. Its liquid content also helps in the natural detoxification process as it aids in washing out toxins from the body. Regular consumption of fruits also speeds up digestion because of its dietary fiber. And this type of produce is not only nutritious, but it also carries antioxidant properties that make the body resistant to certain forms of diseases (cancer, heart problems, etc.).

The most popular types of fruits that are used in detox programs include lemons, oranges, and limes. These citrus fruits are rich in Vitamin C and they stimulate an enzymatic process that promotes proper functioning of the digestive system. Lemon juice, in particular, is often used in liver cleansing programs. A few drops of lemon extract is mixed with a glass of warm water and taken in first thing in the morning. Its Vitamin C properties act as a detox agent, and toxic materials are transformed into digestible substances.

Vegetables

It is also important that **vegetables** are included in one's regular diet. These are best consumed in their raw form as the nutrients are preserved that way. Green veggies are considered to be the most nutritious type, so including kale, spinach, parsley, and other leafy vegetables in your recipes is highly recommended.

The chlorophyll content of green produce is also particularly good for the immune system as it helps fight environmental stresses. Aside from the smog and pollution that can be inhaled through the air, we are also constantly exposed to pesticides, cleaning products, herbicides, and heavy metals. That's why this diet is usually adapted by individuals who are on a liver detox program.

Natural detoxification of the digestive system can also be accomplished through regular intake of garlic and broccoli. Garlic stimulates the liver so that it produces enzymes that will assist the filtering process when the food passes through the digestive tract. Broccoli, on the other hand, is high in antioxidants, and live enzymes in the digestive system are stimulated to promote proper digestion and regular bowel movement.

You can also juice a mixture of different vegetables so as to make a nutritious tonic drink. Adding carrots, cabbages, cauliflower, and asparagus to a juice recipe creates a foundation for an efficient cleansing process.

Green Tea

Tea drinks have also been used as healing treatment since ancient times. And **Green Tea** in particular is known to carry high doses of antioxidants. Its water content is essential in flushing out toxic wastes, and the antioxidant known as Catechins promotes proper functioning of the liver to aid in the detoxification process.

Mung Beans

As Mung beans are easy to digest, these are often included in detox dietary programs. Because of its high fiber content, it can absorb toxic residue that are stored along the linings of the intestinal walls.

All types of beans are high in dietary fiber, and this promotes regular bowel movement. And as we all know, this is the body's natural way of releasing toxic elements from the system. Being able to eliminate waste products regularly also helps in avoiding the development of diseases in the stomach area as toxic materials are eliminated from the body before they can harden up.

Seeds and Nuts

Seeds and nuts are highly digestible, and they supply the body with protein during an intense detox program. The most nutritious nuts and seeds include sunflower seeds, almonds, flax seeds, walnuts, and sesame seeds.

Omega 3 Oil

Omega 3 oils are very nutritious and they coat the lining of the intestines to prevent toxic wastes from sticking to its walls. Likewise, harmful substances are also absorbed by the oil so that these can be eliminated from the body through the lymphatic system.

Grains

The body needs food products that are sourced from grains as this provides for energy and strength. However, brown rice is preferred over white rice as this has gone through less processing. Likewise, whole wheat bread is also healthier than white bread.

Brown rice and wheat bread are often used during the process of breaking off a fast. These are easy to digest, and the body is not immediately exposed to hard solid food. Just keep in mind that it is always best to take in light and small portions of meals at a time. Heavy meals that are consumed in large quantities can force the digestive system to work double time, and malfunction in the process.

Starting a Water Detox Therapy

Ion Detox Water Therapy

Ion detox water therapy is popular to those who are seeking an easy, safe, and non-evasive type of detox program. This method works by removing toxins from the major organs of the body (gall bladder, liver, kidneys) through the pores on the feet. This procedure is best done in a spa as they have all the instruments, gadgets, and treatment solutions that are necessary to make the system effective.

An ion detox machine is needed for this type of method as positive and negative ions need to be produced. The feet should then be soaked on the machine for about 30 minutes to allow the electrical ions to enter the body.

As the positive and negative ions attach themselves to the toxic elements that are present in the system, these are pulled out of the body. That's why you will notice a change in the color of the water mixture in the basin as the waste materials can make it look blurred and muddy.

The process of osmosis also takes place in this method of detox, and this neutralizes the presence of toxic elements inside the body. This makes it easier for the internal organs to release toxins from the system and self-cleanse naturally.

Water Fasting Detox Therapy

Water is essential to life, and you can also use this as an effective means of detoxifying the body naturally. You can fast for several days if you want to give your body a break from always consuming unhealthy types of food. But as this form of fasting limits your nutritional intake, it may render the body weak and susceptible to diseases. For this reason, it is advised that ample rest is taken during the program, and that only light work is included in one's daily routine.

As with all types of fasting, solid food should be gradually introduced to the body. Soft diet that mainly includes fruits and vegetables is recommended, and these should be juiced, steamed, or taken in soup form. One's normal diet can return in a few days when the system has already adjusted to the intake of semi-solid food.

What Should You Drink in the Morning Before You Eat Anything?

Maintaining a healthy body requires proper functioning of all internal organs. In order to assist the process, you can do your part by keeping these organs clean and detoxified from harmful substances. There are particular drinks that you can take in the morning to achieve this goal.

Lemon Juice

Squeezing lemon extracts in a glass of warm water will provide you with a refreshing drink in the morning. This mixture also has a detoxifying and alkalizing effect so that it balances out the body's chemistry and makes it resistant to illnesses.

This particular concoction is also commonly used in weight loss programs as it stimulates the enzymes in the digestive system to speed up digestion. The same process also encourages regular bowel movement so that waste products are expelled from the body before they can stick to the walls of the intestines and harden up.

Consuming lemon juice as a detox concoction requires that the drink is taken in first thing in the morning. This is not consumed with meals, but is rather taken in one go to get one's desired results.

This type of lemon juice drink also activates the gall bladder so that it can efficiently release stored toxic elements from the previous day. To make the system work, this should be consumed at least 30 minutes before a meal.

A few drops of lemon in a glass of water will also benefit the heart, liver, lungs and kidneys. It oxygenates the blood so that oxygen is transported to all the major organs of the body efficiently. Aside from promoting proper functioning of the liver in its filtering job, it also aids in breaking down calcium deposits that are trapped in the kidneys.

As with all citrus fruits, lemons are also rich in Vitamin C, and this helps in neutralizing the negative effects of free radicals in the environment that can damage the healthy cells of the body. Cholesterol build-up is also prevented as it promotes proper elimination of harmful substances through the lymphatic system.

Only those with advanced kidney disorders need to be wary of taking in this lemon juice concoction. Certain types of diseases make this type of fruit intolerable, and it can worsen one's health condition and even put a person's life at risk. That's why it is always important to seek medical advice before adapting any form of detox procedure.

Water

As simple as it may sound, water is the best type of drink that you can consume before you eat anything in the morning. It is safe for everyone, and it is also readily available.

Two to four glasses of water taken in before any type of beverage or food is found to be good for the body in general. It prepares the digestive system for the whole day's food consumption by stimulating the glands on the stomach walls.

The introduction of water early on in the system also hydrates the kidneys so that it can flush out toxins from the body effectively. Likewise, this element can also soften the hardened fecal waste matter in the colon so these can be expelled naturally and regularly. This helps in the prevention of intestinal diseases as hardened bowel contains toxic elements.

How Much Apple Cider Should You Take to Detoxify Your Body?

Even small doses of apple cider vinegar can be beneficial to the body. It contains high amounts of vitamins and minerals especially in its raw and unprocessed form.

Putting in one to three teaspoons of apple cider vinegar in a glass of water is particularly helpful to the digestive system especially when taken in before a meal. It prepares the stomach for the intake of food and speeds up digestion as well.

Apple cider vinegar also aids in liver detox as it purifies the blood and stimulates proper circulation of oxygen to the entire body. And since it also carries live enzymes, it helps in the process of detoxification and cleansing as well.

The acidic compounds in this type of vinegar also help in fighting off bacteria and fungi that can weaken the body's immune system. And when combined with a healthy lifestyle that includes regular exercises and proper diet, the body becomes less susceptible to diseases.

There are other variations to the use of apple cider vinegar too. You can also add a teaspoon of honey to the mixture of water and apple cider vinegar so as to make the concoction even more nutritious. And as honey also contains antioxidant properties, the drink becomes totally cleansing.

Because of its generally pleasant taste, apple cider vinegar can also be added to food recipes. It is frequently added to sauces and salad dressings, and it can be liberally used without fear of any harmful side effects or overdose.

Apple cider vinegar in conjunction with Epsom salt can even be used in cleansing baths. Mixing a cup of apple cider vinegar and a cup of Epsom salt to a hot bath can be very soothing for the body. The solution works by drawing out toxic substances from the body and releasing these through the pores of the skin. This is a great way to jumpstart the process of cleansing, and it can be practiced while undergoing other forms of detox programs too.

When used as a cleansing bath, apple cider vinegar is said to improve one's skin condition by getting rid of acne, and it can also treat other skin problems like eczema and psoriasis. Joint pain and muscle pain can also be relieved as the hot bath solution can also soothe the entire body.

Is the Maple Syrup and Cayenne Pepper Diet Really Effective for Body Detox?

Maple syrup and cayenne pepper are added to lemon juice when a person goes through the **Master Cleanse** method. A typical recipe requires 2 tablespoons of lemon juice, 1 tablespoon of maple syrup, a pinch of cayenne pepper, and 8 ounces of purified water. This cleansing diet can be carried on for about 10 days, and it can be practiced once a year for detoxification purposes. However, if the method is adapted as a weight loss program, a longer period of time may be needed (up to 14 days).

The maple syrup and cayenne pepper diet requires that a person consumes 6 to 12 glasses of the concoction every day. While engaged in this program, you are not allowed to take in any other food or beverages. As this is considered to be an intense form of liquid diet, you should seek the guidance of a physician during the program.

This cleansing formula is said to be effective in organ cleansing as it aids in the proper flushing out of toxic matter from the body. Excess water is also purged out of the system so as to reduce bloating and swelling. A congested liver can also be cleansed so that it can filter the harmful chemicals inside the body efficiently.

The combination of water, lemon extracts, maple syrup, and cayenne pepper is a great energy-booster as well-functioning organs can bring about an efficient cleansing system that revitalizes the whole body. You may, however, experience having headaches, loose stools, and even acne as the system goes through the cleansing process.

Chapter 5: Healthy and Effective Herbal Supplements for Body Detox

Green Tea for Body Detox

The use of green tea for medicinal purposes has been going on for a thousand years. In ancient times, tea leaves are steeped in boiling water so that its extracted juices can be consumed in liquid form. In today's modern times, however, herbal teas are presented in more convenient forms and there are even those types of tea that can simply be steeped in hot water and immediately consumed.

The popularity of herbal teas can be attributed to its basic contents. Compared to coffee, it contains less amounts of caffeine. This is especially true for **Green Tea** as it is milder than other types of tea drinks.

The healing property of green tea has also been documented in many clinical studies. As this is sourced from unfermented leaves, it is presented in raw form. And as it goes through the least processing methods as compared to other types of herbal teas; it also contains more Polyphenols which is an antioxidant agent.

Other medicinal benefits of **Green Tea** can be attributed to its diuretic effects. This helps in the process of detoxification and can even aid weight loss programs as it eliminates water retention. Furthermore, this type of tea also aids in digestion to speed up the body's metabolism. This will result in the proper elimination of body fat, and cholesterol levels and blood pressure are regulated as well.

You will not overdose from green tea as this is a natural product. However, as this still contains caffeine, people who are over sensitive to said substance should monitor their daily intake of the drink. Typically, 2 to 3 cups of green tea in a day can supply the body with sufficient antioxidants to make it resistant to free radicals. But ample amounts of water should also be included in one's regular regimen.

The free radicals that are constantly present in the environment pose risks to the body as it becomes prone to developing killer diseases like cancer and heart problems. But the antioxidant properties that are contained in **Green Tea** can protect the healthy cells of the body and prevent the free radicals from causing damage to a person's DNA structure.

Although deemed to be highly effective as a detox agent, green tea is not recommended to everyone. Because of its caffeine content, it can prove to be harmful to infants and young children. In fact, even pregnant and nursing mothers are advised against drinking this type of herbal drink.

You should also consult a doctor if you are suffering from some form of heart problem. As caffeine can cause palpitations, it can trigger heart attacks to over-sensitive individuals.

Herbal Detox Bath

As **herbal detox bath** makes use of natural components, it is considered to be safe. However, due to the lack of clinical studies, there are no sufficient evidences that can lead to the conclusion that it really works.

The method requires that the body is soaked in a hot bath filled with water and herbal components that may come in powder form. As the body is immersed in the solution for about 30 minutes, the cleansing agents that are present in the water is gradually absorbed by the skin and carried onto the blood stream.

The process becomes even more efficient when this is combined with a massage session as the skin is stimulated to be more receptive to the herbal elements. Toxic wastes are then pulled out from the body and released through the skin in the form of sweat. And the quality of the water in the bath tub will even transform as it becomes filled with waste products that are expelled from the system.

According to practitioners of this method, it can be compared to taking in herbal medicines as the same components are absorbed by the body. The same effects can also be expected, so one will feel relaxed right after the herbal detox bath.

This method can also be held in conjunction with weight loss programs. It lessens the stresses of an intensive detox program, and can even alleviate certain side effects that are attributed to such cleansing methods.

Herbal detox baths have also been reported to be anti-inflammatory, anti-fungal, and anti-stress.

Supplements to Detoxify Your Body

Herbal detox capsules can now be easily purchased and taken in even without prescription. Those who are going through stress-filled days usually resort to this method of detox because of its convenience. By following the directions on the package, a person can typically take in the herbal capsules a few times in a day.

This type of supplement is also known for its benefits to the digestive system. As constipation can lead to a lot of stomach problems, having regular bowel movement becomes of utmost importance. If one is low on fiber-intake, herbal capsules can often help in regulating daily elimination of waste products.

Herbal supplements can restore and balance the chemical composition of the body. And as these can boost one's metabolism, all the major organs of the body can function properly. Calories are even burned faster, so the method is also effective as a support system to weight loss programs.

Natural ingredients are used in herbal supplements to make it safe and effective as well. Some of the commonly used herbs include basil, fennel, parsley, and celery. The basil content particularly benefits the heart, bladder, and brain as it promotes the production and proper circulation of oxygen.

When a supplement contains fennel, it would be particularly helpful in losing weight. This ingredient can control hunger and food cravings, and it even has diuretic effects. The antimicrobial properties of this type of herb also aid in making the body strong and resistant to disease-causing germs.

The parsley component of a supplement also supplies the body with natural antibiotic properties. Infections are treated and prevented, and toxic substances are also flushed out of the system through the kidneys. And as with the raw form of parsley, this ingredient is known to be helpful in regulating one's blood pressure as well as in keeping the digestive tract well-functioning.

If the herbal detox capsule contains celery, it becomes a blood purifier and cleanser too. Celery is said to be good in alleviating the symptoms of fatigue, and it also reduces intestinal problems as it speeds up digestion. This type of herb also carries B complex vitamins which can aid in rheumatism problems. And it helps in the detox process by assisting in the excretion of waste materials too.

It is highly advised that water intake is increased when one is taking herbal detox supplements. This will aid in flushing out the system from toxic substances so that the body can be cleansed more efficiently. If carried on properly, taking detoxifying supplements can improve one's skin condition and increase the body's energy and stamina as well.

Are Supplements for Body Detox Safe and Effective?

Body detox supplements that contain natural ingredients are generally safe and effective as they carry the same results as the raw ingredients. These can be nourishing as well as cleansing as the organs of the body are supplied with all the essential vitamins and minerals that promote natural expulsion of toxic substances.

You should be careful, however, as to the type of supplements that you take as not all body detox medications are sourced from natural ingredients. And sometimes, even if the contents are taken from natural sources, the process of production may render the supplements ineffective.

When supplements are made to undergo too much heat during processing, some of the essential nutrients may evaporate. Furthermore, some methods of processing may involve the use of chemical substances, and this will ultimately reduce the nutritional value of the tablets or capsules. In fact, having chemical contents can even make a detox supplement dangerous as it introduces more toxic substances to the system.

It is therefore advised that due care is exercised when deciding to take detox supplements, and that the package labels are read meticulously. Asking for medical advice will also safeguard one's health as a medical practitioner will know which supplements are beneficial to your condition.

Chapter 6: Simple Tips on How to Start an Effective Detox Program for Your Body

Preparation before a Body Detox

Preparation for detoxification is important if you want to make the system really effective and beneficial to your health. Otherwise, you will only be wasting your time, effort, and money as the program will not work efficiently.

See a Doctor

You should consult a doctor before undergoing any type of program that affects your health and body. This way, your condition can be evaluated properly in order to find out if you can handle the stresses and side effects that are associated with certain types of detox program. This is especially important if you intent to carry out a program for an extended period of time as it can put your health at risk.

Make a Plan

First of all, you need to prepare for a detox program by abstaining from caffeine, salt, sugar, and other forms of preservatives. Solid foods, especially those that are fatty and oily, need to be avoided too. And if you really want to make the program successful, alcoholic beverages as well as cigarettes need to be removed from one's lifestyle.

If you are on medication, it may be necessary to stop taking the prescribed drugs temporarily while on a body detox program. This will ensure that your medicines will not interfere with the system of detoxification that you have chosen to adapt. However, you should get a clearance from your physician first, as refraining from the intake of prescription drugs may be prove to be dangerous to your health condition.

Practice Discipline

As a detox program can be quite intense, you need to discipline yourself and set realistic goals. Aside from physical preparation, you also need to prepare your body mentally and emotionally. You may experience having food cravings when going through certain methods of detox (e.g. water fasting, juice fasting, etc.) and your mind should be strong enough to resist the urge to eat. Furthermore, side effects like irritability and moodiness can also be expected, as the body is going through a system of cleansing and detoxifying.

Get Enough Rest

The body can be weak and vulnerable while undergoing the detox process. Because of this, ample rest is required in order to preserve the body's energy. Although you can still carry out your regular routines, 8 hours of sleep is recommended.

Sleeping is the best form of healing, and this will aid the detox program by making the system more efficient. Even afternoon naps can rejuvenate the body and supply it with the needed energy to carry out the remaining tasks of the day.

Light Exercises

If losing weight is your main goal for undergoing a detox procedure, adapting exercise routines will make the system more effective. However, at this time, only light exercises are recommended as vigorous workout routines can be too hard and demanding for the body. Yoga, Pilates, and simple exercises like walking and climbing the stairs are sufficient at this point in a detox program.

Follow the Directions on the Package

If you decide to take on detox supplements and pills, you should read the package directions first. Not doing so may result in an unsuccessful detox method as you may be taking the supplements on a wrong dosage. Taking in less than the recommended dosage may render the supplements ineffective, and taking too much can result in an overdose and put your health and even your life at risk.

Physical Preparation for a Detox Bath

Should you decide to adapt a detox procedure by going on a cleansing bath, the body should be cleaned first. Scrubbing and exfoliating before the actual detox bath will unclog the pores on the skin so that the herbal solution can be readily absorbed by the skin. Likewise, the elimination of waste matter is also more successful as the toxins are drawn out of the skin more efficiently.

Activities to Avoid While Undergoing Body Detox

In general, strenuous activities should be avoided while undergoing a body detox program. As the body releases toxins and waste products from the system, you may feel weak as the body lacks the needed energy to carry out vigorous activities.

If you are regularly exercising, you may still continue to do so, but only mild forms of workout routines are recommended. At this point, it is not advisable to lift weights and perform similar types of exercises. Only walking, jogging, and other similar forms of workout methods that are not too demanding for the body are allowed.

The chores and activities that you can do while doing a body detox will largely depend on your stamina and overall health condition, so it is important to listen to your body. If you choose to adapt an intensive detox program, it is only necessary that you try to conserve your energy in order to be able to finish the system successfully.

Going on a water fast, for example, can deplete the body of energy. So you should take as much rest as possible. In fact, this method typically requires bed rest as the body is cut from its source of nutrients and may feel weak and vulnerable to illnesses.

You can take on normal activities if you go on a less demanding form of body detox like juice fasting. As you are consuming fruit and vegetable extracts in this type of program, the body is still supplied with the basic nutrients that it needs to function normally. However, it will still depend on how your body adjusts to the program as it can also carry some side effects.

If you are experiencing loose bowel movement, it is only natural that you avoid doing activities and chores that require the use of too much energy and effort. Having loose stools can cause dehydration, and this will deplete the body of strength and stamina. That's why it is also recommended that drinking water (at least 8 glasses a day) is incorporated in this program as it will not only aid in flushing out toxins, but will also help in keeping the body well-hydrated.

One should not assume that taking on a less demanding form of cleansing method like taking detox pills is less stressful for the body. Although this type of detox is not that mentally challenging, it still exposes the body to certain forms of side effects. The body may feel weak, and you may also experience having gas and other stomach problems.

Perhaps the only type of detox that won't present any serious side effect is going on a cleansing bath. This method is known to be soothing and relaxing, and it doesn't result in feeling weak too. However, like ionic foot bath, the program is quite questionable as to its effectiveness in cleansing the body. And as both types of methods have not gone through enough research, we cannot conclude that they really work in eliminating toxins from the body.

Are there People Who Should Not Undergo a Body Detox?

Because of the side effects that are commonly associated with detox programs, it is not considered to be safe for everyone. There are certain types of people and conditions that should be carefully assessed before attempting to go through certain detox programs.

Pregnant and Nursing Women

Women who are pregnant need to take care of themselves and their babies as well. As the fetus is still connected to the mother, anything the mom does will affect the baby directly. This is especially true with food and medicinal intake, so one should really be careful as to what enters the system as it can pose health risks to the baby inside the womb.

The same holds true for nursing mothers as the infant's supply of milk passes through the mother's system. Medicinal residues as well as chemicals from food taken in are all present in the blood stream, and these can pass on to the child as he or she is being nursed and breastfed.

Another reason why pregnant and nursing mothers should refrain from undergoing a detox program is that a particular method may hinder the supply of the needed nutrients of a developing baby. Calcium and protein are particularly in high demand when the body is carrying a baby. And cleansing programs like fasting will expose the body to very limited supply of vitamins and minerals.

Babies and Children

Compared to adults, babies and children require more nutrients to assist in their growth and development. Aside from bone structure, the internal organs are not yet fully developed at a very young age. For this reason, babies and children are not supposed to undergo a system that will limit the supply of essential vitamins and minerals that are needed by the body. Doing so may result in stunted growth and other forms of abnormalities. Furthermore, underdeveloped organs will make the body weak and prone to diseases.

People with Serious Medical Conditions

While cleansing programs may be helpful to people who are suffering from serious ailments. Due care and precaution should also be taken. Seeking a doctor's advice is strongly recommended in order to ensure one's safety.

Diabetes

Those who have **diabetes** should have their conditions examined first before undergoing any form of detox method. As the blood sugar levels of diabetics are very sensitive, any imbalance in the system may prove to be fatal. This is especially true if one chooses to go on a fast, whether water fasting or juice fasting.

Water fasting can cause an imbalance in the system which could lead to fluctuations of the blood sugar level. And this is detrimental to one's health as it could lead to complications like heart attack and stroke.

And even if you choose to go on a juice diet, this is also not a guarantee of safety. You see, there are certain types of produce that can cause the sugar levels to rise and fall (e.g. grapefruits), so these should be avoided. Moreover, the limited intake of food can also cause an imbalance in the system which is extremely dangerous if one is diabetic.

Heart Problems

As with those suffering from diabetes, people with heart problems should also be careful with the cleansing methods that they adapt. Although these types of programs are generally beneficial for the heart, the intensity of the program may prove to be too demanding for a weak heart.

A sudden change in the diet and daily routines can influence the condition of the heart. It can cause palpitations, and a person may even experience difficulty in breathing. These conditions can trigger a heart attack, and it can also lead to other complications like stroke and increased sugar levels.

Cancer

Cancer patients should be particularly cautious about the methods that are undertaken when one attempts to detoxify the body. This health condition requires utmost care as any forms of stress can aggravate the situation. Dieting and engaging in strenuous activities need to be carefully monitored as not doing so can put one's life at risk.

As the body is extremely sensitive when there are cancer cells in the system, nutritious food is very much needed by the body. As such, a detox method like water fasting should be avoided as this form of cleansing limits the body of essential vitamins and minerals. It would greatly help if the intake of foods that are filled with chemicals and preservatives is avoided as these can lead to further multiplication of cancer cells.

Likewise, you should also consult a doctor if you are considering going on a juice diet. Even if the system provides for nutrients, the method itself can still be too demanding for one suffering from cancer. As the internal organs go through a detoxification process, it can be quite stressful physically and mentally. And stressful situations can be fatal for cancer patients as the internal organs become overburdened with the adrenaline flow.

Eating Disorders

Some forms of body detox are not advisable to be undertaken by those who have eating disorders. Fasting and dieting, in particular, can cause chemical imbalance and further worsen the condition. Or even if one has already recuperated from the illness, a sudden change in the food intake can bring back the problem again.

It is always wise to see a doctor before attempting to undergo any change in the diet. And those with eating disorders, or anorexic, need to be particularly cautious so as not to endanger one's life.

Under Medication

If you are currently being treated of a medical condition and are using prescription drugs, a detox procedure may not be advisable for you. Engaging in an intense method of cleansing may have an adverse effect on your prescribed medicines, and the drugs may also hinder the effectiveness of the procedure.

You should ask your physician if it is indeed safe and practical to take on a detox program while undergoing medication. And your doctor can make the necessary recommendation as to whether to go through a cleansing procedure at the moment or not. It might even be more practical to stop taking the medicines for a while until the detox program is completed.

What Should You Eat After a Body Detox?

You should definitely not go back to eating meat products and fatty foods right after completing a body detox, especially if you have gone through several days of fasting. Doing so will result in stomach upset and chemical imbalance, as the sudden intake of solid food will disturb the system.

The best types of food to take right after fasting are fruits and vegetables, and it is also better if these are organic. If you have fasted for about a week or so, you should still be on a soft diet. At this point, steamed veggies, broths, and salads can be taken in small amounts. You can then gradually eat whole fruits and raw vegetables gradually.

Although you can already start eating solid food like beef, pork, and chicken when your system has already adjusted to solid foods, you should avoid recipes that contain too many preservatives. Likewise, greasy food should also be taken in small amounts so as not to clog the system again.

If you are fond of eating rice with your meals, you should consume brown rice instead of white rice. Brown rice is more nutritious as it has gone through less processing, and it is easier to digest too.

As much as possible, you should drink caffeinated drinks like coffee and tea sparingly. It is also much better to stick to freshly squeezed fruit and vegetable juices rather than buy commercially produced drinks from the store as these can contain chemicals and preservatives. Your daily intake of water should also be around 8 glasses, as keeping the body well-hydrated aids in detoxifying the body naturally through urinating and sweating.

If you want to maintain the positive results that you have gotten from a detox procedure, focusing on your diet should be one of your main goals. By eating only food products like fruits and veggies, you can provide the body with a natural source of vitamins and minerals. Eating meat products, on the other hand, should be done sparingly.

How Long Should You Do Your First Body Detox Diet?

First timers should not attempt to go on a body detox diet for a very long period of time. As the system is new and unfamiliar, it can cause trauma and undue suffering when not carried out properly. This is especially true for fasting programs as these methods can be very demanding and challenging.

You can test the system by trying on a detox diet for a few days. One to three days is often recommended for beginners as said time frame can give you an idea as to how the system feels like. You can then make a decision as to whether you'd want to carry on the program for a longer period the next time around.

You can also go on a series of short fasts as you are trying to adjust to the method. You can then add a day or two to your succeeding fasts as you get adjusted to the system. As long as your body can handle the procedure, it would be generally safe for your health. That's why you should learn to listen to your body, and simply discontinue the program if it proves to be too uncomfortable and painful.

Typically, a one-week fast is recommended either as a maintenance procedure or as regular means of cleansing the system. Because the entire procedure is carried on for several days, toxic elements are flushed out of the system gradually. As harmful waste materials are eliminated slowly from the body, it will not disturb the normal functioning of the internal organs.

Still, the best way to know how long a body detox diet should last is to ask your doctor about it. As the condition of every individual differs from one another, so does the recommended amount of time that should be devoted to a diet procedure.

Chapter 7: Dr. Oz's 2-Day Detox Program

Who is Dr. Oz and How Does His 2-Day Cleansing Program Work?

Dr. Mehmet Oz of the Dr. Oz Show is a well-known doctor (surgeon), author of health-related books, and TV personality. He was featured on the Oprah Winfrey show, and this added to his already growing popularity. Millions of viewers became impressed with the 2-day cleansing program that he invented, and a lot of people wanted to try the method out immediately.

Dr. Oz's detox program is not like any other methods that call for strict diet and starvation. In fact, you can eat satisfying meals while undergoing the procedure, and even take in an unlimited portion of the allowed snacks.

While the system doesn't promise that you will lose weight as a result of the program, it guarantees that your body will be cleansed from toxic substances. During the 48-hour detox method, the live enzymes inside your body will be stimulated so that these can efficiently breakdown the toxic elements in your system. And as the procedure also promotes proper functioning of all the major organs in your body, waste products can be flushed out effectively.

According to Dr. Oz, his method is safer and more useful than traditional detox systems that only aim to lose weight. If this is the only goal for a detox program, the body's natural metabolism may be affected and even damaged. You see, while it is possible to lose as much as 20 pounds in as short as 2 weeks, it may pose some health risks to the body. Abrupt changes in one's diet can ruin the natural flow of digestion and elimination, and this can result in a messed-up system. And when this happens, all the extra pounds that you lost in just a short period of time can come back as soon as you start eating normally again as the body's metabolism has slowed down considerably.

With Dr. Oz's cleansing and detox program, however, the body is supplied with all the necessary nutrients needed for proper digestion and elimination. The meals and snacks in this system promote enzyme activity, and this will not only result in detoxification but in well-nourished organs as well.

The 2-day program is recommended to be carried out 3 to 4 times a year or whenever you feel sluggish and out of energy. The method is capable of rejuvenating the body so that one will feel in sync physically and mentally again. You can even take on this method if you feel bloated as it is also effective in eliminating the symptoms of water retention. By nourishing the lungs, liver, colon, and kidneys, excess water as well as harmful substances can be efficiently flushed out of the body.

Dr. Oz's Breakfast Recipe – Quinoa with Dried Prunes

During the 2-day detox program, Dr. Oz suggests eating a breakfast which consists of a bowl of Quinoa mixed in with some prunes. This whole grain meal is full of amino acids, and it's a good source of protein as well. It is way better than other cleansing programs as other methods restrict the diet of protein sources, and this can be quite harmful for the body.

The lack of needed protein can push the system to get its source from the muscle tissues which can result in the decrease of muscle mass. And as we all know, weight watchers aim to shed off pounds by losing fat, and not muscle mass.

This hearty breakfast is also filling as the prunes are high in fiber. Moreover, this component has a laxative effect, so it helps in promoting regular bowel movement as well.

Dr. Oz's Lunch Recipe – Delicious and Natural Fruit Smoothie

Dr. Oz suggests taking in a delicious and satisfying fruit smoothie for lunch. By combining blueberries, bananas, and flaxseed in a blender or juicer, you will be provided with a very nutritious and filling meal.

Like all the other fruits in the berry family, blueberries contain high levels of antioxidants. It particularly carries a component called Quercetin which promotes enzyme production in the liver. This element is also capable of neutralizing the damaging effects of free radicals in the environment.

Banana is also popular in dieting and detoxification methods; and this can be taken in whole form or juiced form. For this particular meal, however, the banana ingredient is mixed with other ingredients to create a smoothie recipe. The program benefits from this component as bananas are loaded with B6. This B vitamin can boost the performance of the detoxifying enzymes within the body so that toxic substances can be flushed out of the system properly.

The addition of grounded flaxseeds in the mixture not only adds some distinct taste to the recipe but it provides for an additional source of fiber as well. Fiber is very much needed in getting rid of chemical waste products particularly in the colon area, as this component acts as a broom in sweeping away harmful materials from the walls of the intestines.

Dr. Oz's Dinner Recipe – Vegetable Broth, Sauerkraut, and Sliced Apples

The main meal for dinner is comprised of a soup that's loaded with very nutritious vegetables. Simply combine some garlic, cabbage, fennel, parsley, shiitake mushrooms, and cayenne pepper in a pot, add some water, and simmer the mixture over medium heat. For best results, the vegetables should not be overcooked as they can lose some of the vitamins and minerals contained therein.

The garlic component in this recipe acts as an antioxidant; it is also widely known as a natural antibiotic as it helps the body in fighting against bacteria. Cabbage is a perfect source for B complex, so it works in soothing the nerves and providing the system with energy especially at this time of detoxification.

Fennel promotes the secretion of bile, and this method assists in flushing waste matter from the liver. Parsley adds a familiar taste to the broth; and as this ingredient is considered to be diuretic, it helps in releasing toxic substances through the urine.

By adding in shiitake mushrooms to the mixture, the soup becomes a more potent meal. This type of mushroom has high nutritional value that can strengthen the immune system, and it also has anti-viral properties. This ingredient is also commonly included in weight loss programs as it helps in regulating the body's cholesterol levels and blood pressure. That's why including shiitake mushroom in a soup is also beneficial if one aims to undergo a detox procedure.

The last ingredient to be included in the recipe is the cayenne pepper. This is another common component in weight loss and detox recipes. The main purpose of adding this to the mixture is that it stimulates the live enzymes present in the lungs so that this organ can expel poisonous gases from the system efficiently. And of course, it also has a distinct taste that makes a soup more delicious and interesting.

Dr. Oz also allows some side dishes to go with this soup. You can take some fermented Sauerkraut with this meal as this contains probiotic components. Said element is responsible for breaking down toxic substances that are present in the intestines so that these can be properly eliminated through bowel movement.

Some slices of apple are also included in the dinner recipe as treat, and the added fiber contained in the fruit further facilitates colon cleansing. And having a good source of vitamin C is also helpful to the entire method as this is a great immunity booster.

Dr. Oz's Snack Recipe – Pineapple, Kale and Artichoke Juice

For the snack, Dr. Oz combines pineapple, kale, and artichoke to make a delicious and nutritious juice. You can prepare this either in a blender or a juicer, whichever you prefer. While some people choose to use a blender so that even the pulp and fiber can be processed, there are also those who prefer a juicer because it produces less heat while processing the ingredients. Too much heat can result in the evaporation of vital nutrients, and it therefore decreases the nutritional value of the drink.

This snack can be taken as much as you like all throughout the 48-hour cleansing method as it will not hinder the process of detoxification. However, it is recommended that that at least 2 glasses of the prepared juice is consumed in between meals.

The pineapple component in this juice activates the enzymes in the digestive system. Because of this, there will be proper digestion and absorption of nutrients from food products.

Kale is also an important ingredient in this recipe as it supports the production of enzymes in the liver. This allows the organ to filter toxic substances more efficiently so that the body will not be burdened by too many harmful chemicals.

And adding in artichoke to the juice recipe aids in improving bile flow to reduce the risk of constipation. By having regular bowel movement, especially while carrying out a cleansing procedure, your system will be more receptive to the benefits of detoxification.

Advantages of Adapting Dr. Oz's 2-Day Body Detox Method

Dr. Oz's detox method is quite interesting as it mainly involves the consumption of whole foods. Moreover, it doesn't require the practitioner to starve one's self in order to attain favorable results. As a matter of fact, the snack recipe can even be consumed as often as you like.

A lot of people will also find this method easy to carry out as it only requires 2 days for full detoxification. The system can therefore be performed over the weekend wherein one is not preoccupied with work. This makes the program not only more achievable but less stressful as well.

As with almost all types of detox and weight loss programs, note that this program also necessitates frequent trips to the toilet. While it is only normal to have recurrent cases of bowel movements, the stools are supposed to be normal and not loose. The body is merely eliminating waste materials from the system so that the whole body will feel rejuvenated and revitalized again.

This method is also good for losing weight, although it is not the sole purpose of the system. By allowing all the vital organs in the body to function properly, your metabolism will also speed up so that stored fat can be shed off easily. So if you are currently undergoing a weight loss program, you can adapt this detox method as a supplemental procedure to enhance its overall effects to your body.

According to Dr. Oz, finishing the 48-hour detox method will make you feel good again. As your body is cleansed from the inside out, the burden of having toxic build-up will be greatly reduced if not totally eliminated.

Some Key Pointers on How to Make the Most of Dr. Oz's 2-Day Cleansing Program

The Importance of Water

As with all cleansing methods, drinking plenty of water is encouraged when taking on this program. Water helps in flushing out harmful substances from the body, so this will make the system more effective.

Sleep is Essential for Success

It has always been said that the human body needs at least 8 hours of sleep in a day. When the body is at rest, all the major organs can take a break too. If you are currently involved in a detox procedure, your body will need as much rest as it can get. This way, the system can work more efficiently in expelling toxic substances from the body when one is awake.

Refrain from Eating After 7PM

In order to encourage proper digestion, you need to let your digestive system rest before falling asleep. It takes about 1 to 2 hours to fully digest a meal, that's why it is strongly advised that the last meal or snack you take be done before 7PM. This way, you can go to bed early and complete your 8 hours of sleep.

Warm Bath with Epsom Salt

You can dissolve 2 cups of Epsom salt in the bathtub for a soothing bath before retiring at night. The Epsom salt contains large doses of magnesium which can be absorbed by the body through the skin's pores. This element will trigger the release of hundreds of beneficial enzymes inside the body. It's the perfect supplement for many types of detox procedures.

Dandelion Tea before Bed Time

Drinking a cup of dandelion tea before retiring at night is also highly recommended by Dr. Oz. This type of tea is diuretic, so it will stimulate urination in order to release toxins out of the body before going to sleep. Remaining toxic chemicals in the system will also be flushed out when you wake up in the morning.

Chapter 8: The 21-Day Clean Diet Program

How Does the Clean Diet Program Work?

Dr. Alejandro Junger, a New York cardiologist, designed the 21-day clean diet program. As one of the leaders in integrative medicine, he knows how to deal with chronic symptoms of headaches, allergies, depression, irritable bowel syndrome, weight problems, fatigue, insomnia, and other ailments.

According to Dr. Junger, all these health problems can be traced to having accumulated toxins inside the body. But with the proper detox approach, the body can recuperate and heal itself.

Basically, this program requires 21 days to complete. You are to consume liquid meals for breakfast as well as for dinner. For lunch, you are to eat a solid meal. Whole fruits and nuts can be eaten as snacks in between meals.

The Clean Diet Breakfast Suggestions

Some examples of ingredients that you can use for breakfast include mangoes, pineapples, blueberries, raspberries, apples, carrots, broccoli and asparagus. You can juice the aforementioned ingredients or create smoothies with them.

The Clean Diet Lunch Suggestions

As you are allowed to eat a solid meal for lunch, you can cook brown rice and accompany this with lean lamb, chicken, duck, turkey, or any (cold water) fish variety. Steamed or boiled recipes are recommended as you are trying to avoid fatty foods while detoxifying the body.

The Clean Diet Dinner Suggestions

For dinner, you are to consume another liquid meal. You can use the same recipes that you had for breakfast, and drink fresh juices and smoothies. Or if you want, you can cook up some soup. Some of the ingredients that you can use for soup include asparagus, broccoli, spinach, lettuce, and cabbage. All these veggies contain dietary fiber which promotes regular bowel movement.

The Clean Diet Snack Suggestions

You can snack on some raw almonds in between meals so as to keep hunger pangs at bay. You also have the option of eating whole fruits like apples, pears, strawberries, watermelon, and grapes. The fiber and water contents of these fruits help in proper digestion of food and elimination of wastes.

Things to Remember When Going Through the 21-Day Clean Diet Program

1. While you can interchange the lunch and dinner recipes as suggested in the program, it is not that recommendable. You see, the digestive system will have a hard time digesting solid food at night while the body is at rest, and this is counter-productive to a detox plan.

2. There should be a 12-hour window between dinner and breakfast in order to provide the digestive system ample time to rest.

3. As much as possible, you should only use organic fruits and vegetables when creating or cooking detox recipes. Processed foods should also be avoided as they contain preservatives, additives, and coloring.

4. In order to be able to keep up with the 21-day program, you should create interesting and tasty recipes. As this method allows for the use of a wide variety of ingredients (including meat products), you can take on the system comfortably.

5. Exercise should be included in the detox plan. Even simple exercises like walking and taking the stairs whenever possible will do the body good. Sweating is one of the most effective ways of releasing bodily toxins, and the act of exercising will also stimulate proper functioning of all the vital organs in the body. This is also good for cardiovascular health.

6. As you are aiming to cleanse the system of all harmful substances, you should know which types of foods to avoid. In order to reduce the daily load being performed by the digestive system, you should minimize your intake of fatty and greasy food as well as those snacks that are too sweet or salty.

7. Healthy living also plays a major role in cleansing the body. It is therefore advised that alcoholic beverages are avoided as these can slow down the body's natural metabolism. Furthermore, it puts too much work on the liver as this organs works in filtering out the toxic substances that are present in alcohol. Likewise, smoking cigarettes should also be avoided as this makes the lungs work double time in purifying the air that circulates inside the body.

Chapter 9: How the Detox System Really Works

The body's internal organs need to be fully functional in order to avoid certain diseases. When all the major organs in the body are working as they should, one will have optimal health as the body's immune system becomes resistant to germs, bacteria, and pollutants. For this reason, it becomes a necessity to detoxify the body regularly.

Liver Detox

The liver works in allowing nutrients absorbed from food to enter the blood stream so as to nourish the entire body. However, it first filters said nutrients so that contaminants like pesticides, heavy metals (lead, mercury, asbestos, etc) and other toxic substances will not affect the system.

Once filtered, the toxic elements are excreted into bile formation so that all harmful elements can go to the intestines. The waste materials will then be eliminated from the system in the form of stools.

Gall Bladder Detox

Detoxifying the gall bladder goes hand in hand with liver cleansing as this organ is responsible for storing the bile created by the liver. Bile is naturally secreted by the gall bladder right after eating as this allows proper digestion of food products especially the fats.

As diets that are high in fat and cholesterol may prove to be too much for the gall bladder to handle, this can result in the formation of stones. That's why regular detoxification of this organ is necessary from time to time as cleansing the gall bladder can help get rid of such formations.

Through the regular intake of pears, apples, lemon, limes, and seaweeds, gall stone build-up can be avoided. Chamomile tea and flaxseed oil are also commonly included in detox programs to help breakdown and dislodge said stones,

Lung Detox

Lungs serve as air purifiers as they work in filtering out gases, pollution, and particulates that can cause damage to the body. When the lungs are kept healthy and functioning well, they can prevent harmful contaminants from entering and damaging the system.

Kidney Detox

Studies show that the blood circulating through the body is filtered by the kidneys every 35 to 45 minutes. When this organ is detoxified, it will be stimulated to work efficiently in getting rid of toxic elements in the blood stream by releasing these through the process of urination.

Colon Detox

The colon is equipped with a cellular structure that guards this organ from harmful substances. The guarding cells act as soldiers in fighting off toxins from entering into the blood stream.

Through regular bowel movement, chemical wastes, metals, and other poisonous elements are eliminated from the system before they can cause harm to the body. However, this organ needs to be detoxified quite often so that it can function properly. When one takes the colon for granted, there could be a build-up of toxic elements that will be too hard to eliminate.

Blood Detox

It is also important to focus on blood detoxification as this flows through the entire system continuously. It is through the blood that nutrients are distributed all over the body, and it also carries the needed oxygen for the body to function well.

By removing toxic substances from the blood, you are also ensuring that all the vital organs of the body will have improved performance. Aside from increasing the body's resistance and immunity against diseases, you can also avoid having headaches and allergies and eliminate symptoms of fatigue too.

Certain herbs are known to be blood purifiers. Red clover and Burdock root can be included in your cooking recipes as well as juice recipes to benefit from their blood cleansing effects.

Brain Detox

The free radicals that are present in the environment can enter the body and damage the system including the brain. Once your brain neurons are affected, your cognitive senses can decline dramatically. Through detoxification, one can protect the brain cells from being damaged by free radicals, pollution, and other harmful substances that are present not only in the environment but also in the food we eat.

In order to promote proper brain functioning, you can eat brain-enhancing food sources like apples and berries. Apples are known to carry an antioxidant called Quercetin, and this can protect the brain cells from being damaged by toxic elements and free radicals.

Likewise, dark colored berries like blueberries and blackberries are also strongly recommended for daily consumption as these fruits contain a compound called Polyphenols. This compound will safeguard your brain neurons' health so that your mind will stay sharp and alert.

While coffee is not frequently used in detox methods, it is one of the beneficial food sources for the brain. You see, caffeine from coffee beans also carries antioxidants, and these are essential for mental health. In fact, regular intake of coffee has been known to reduce the risk of developing Alzheimer's disease.

Chapter 10: 10 Super-Easy Body Detox Recipes

Detox recipes can come in many forms. As the method calls for limited intake of meals, you need to know the right combination of solid foods that are allowed in the particular program that you are undertaking.

The recipes should be filling and nutritious as you will need strength and stamina to finish the course. So energy booster meals should also be available to help you achieve a successful result.

Listed below are just some of the detox recipes that you can prepare at home. It comprises of meals, snacks, and juices that are easy to make and nutritious as well.

Vegetable with Apple Juice

This tasty recipe is perfect for a detox program, as it is low in fat and high in fiber. It is easy to prepare too, as you simply need to juice the ingredients by using a juicer or a blender.

Although the vegetable ingredients in this type of juice can taste a little awkward, rest assured that it is good for you as celery, beet, and parsley are all high in antioxidant properties. They are therefore the perfect combination of veggies that can help the body fight against the free radicals that exist in the environment.

Adding carrots and apples to the recipe also increases the nutritional value of the drink as these two ingredients are known for their high concentration of Vitamins A and C. The sweet taste of these types of produce can also neutralize the slightly odd-taste of the vegetable components of the juice drink.

Ingredients:

3 Carrots
1 stalk Celery
½ Beet
½ cup Parsley
2 red apples

Procedure:

1. Wash all the ingredients and cut into small pieces.

2. Process all the produce through a juicer or a blender.

3. Consume immediately or serve chilled.

Green Rolls

This recipe is a healthy and filling snack. It can be used in conjunction with cleansing programs, and you can also make it a regular snack even if you are not undergoing a detox procedure. Lettuce is loaded with micronutrients, and it contains high levels of fiber too. Carrots and apples are rich in vitamins A and C. Regular consumption of this type of recipe will therefore refresh you and supply you with essential vitamins and minerals.

Ingredients:

4 Lettuce leaves
1 Carrot
1 Red apple
1 tsp Cayenne pepper

½ cup Non-fat dressing

Procedure:

1. Wash all the ingredients thoroughly and drain off excess water.

2. Cut the carrot and apple into strips.

3. Lay the lettuce leaves flat on a serving dish and put some strips of carrots and apples.

4. Roll the lettuce leaves to hold the carrots and apples inside.

5. Sprinkle with cayenne pepper or top off with non-fat dressing.

Detoxifying Green Juice

While ingredients in this particular recipe are not all colored green, the result will still be green as it will be the dominant color when kale leaves, celery, and parsley are mixed with the rest of the ingredients.

This mixture also involves the use of apple which is high in Vitamin C, and it also contains fiber which is a needed component for cleansing programs. Carrot adds sweetness to the overall taste of the juice and it will also supply you with a high dose of Vitamin A.

As Kale leaf is low in fat, it is a common ingredient in weight loss and cleansing programs. Celery and parsley are commonly used too, as these are both high in fiber and antioxidant properties.

Ingredients:

2 Kale leaves
1 stalk Celery
1 Carrot
1 Apple
½ cup Parsley

Procedure:

1. Wash all the ingredients under running water and drain.

2. Cut the carrot and apple in several chunks to allow for easy processing.

3. Juice all the ingredients in a blender or juicer.

4. Serve cold.

Carrot and Strawberry Juice

Even a simple recipe can be beneficial to a detox program. By combining carrots and strawberries in one delicious juice drink, your body will be provided with vitamins and minerals as well as a source of fiber. This is a perfect snack in between meals as it is filling and refreshing as well.

Ingredients:

5 Carrots
2 cups Strawberries

Procedure:

1. Wash the produce and put on a strainer to get rid of excess water.

2. Cut the carrots in chunks without removing the skin.

3. Process both ingredients in a juicer or blender until the texture is smooth and creamy.

4. Consume immediately and keep the unused portion in the freezer.

Carrot Salad with Sesame Seeds

This recipe is a good addition to cleansing regimens as it is particularly loaded with high-fiber ingredients. Waste products that are trapped inside the body can therefore be released more efficiently as there will be regular bowel movement.

Aside from fiber, this salad also uses carrots and parsley as the main ingredients. So it will also provide you with an abundance of vitamins and minerals. Note too, that this is a simple recipe that you can easily prepare in minutes.

Ingredients:

1 tbsp. Olive oil
1 tbsp Rice Vinegar
1 inch Ginger
¼ tsp. Pepper
3 Carrots
¼ cup Parsley
1 tsp. Sesame seeds

Procedure:
1. Wash all the fruits and vegetables needed for the recipe.

2. Peel and grate the ginger.

3. In a large bowl, combine the grated ginger, olive oil, rice vinegar, and pepper. Whisk all ingredients until well-blended.

4. Put the carrots, parsley, and sesame seeds inside the food processor so as to shred said ingredients.

5. Combine the shredded mixture with the dressing and serve.

Carrot-Apple-Grape Juice

This refreshing juice drink is high in vitamins A, C, and E, so it is also recommended for daily consumption to boost the body's resistance. You will benefit from this detox recipe as the fruits and vegetables mixed herein all contain the much needed fiber that can help eliminate toxic substances from the body.

Ingredients:

3 Carrots
1 Apple
1 cup Grapes

Procedure:
1. Wash all the ingredients thoroughly to make sure that they are free from dirt and pesticides.

2. Cut the apple and carrot in pieces that will fit in your juicer or blender.

3. Put all the ingredients in your juicer or blender to create a delicious juice drink, and serve.

Pure Veggie Juice

If you are an avid juicer, then you will surely love this recipe as it is easy to prepare and nutritious as well. The chlorophyll in the green leafy vegetables carries high levels of antioxidants which can boost the immune system. Carrots will provide you with Vitamin A which is good for the eyes and the skin.

Ingredients:

4 Carrots
4 Lettuce leaves
½ cup Spinach

½ cup Parsley

Procedure:

1. Wash all ingredients and set aside to drain.

2. Cut the carrots in portions that will fit your blender or juicer. Don't remove the skin.

3. Put all the ingredients in the juicer or blender and process until there are no more lumps.

4. Drink at room temperature or chill in the freezer before serving.

Carrot and Potato Soup

This recipe can serve as one of the main meals of the day when undergoing a detox program. The main ingredients are carrots and potatoes which are both highly nutritious crops. Carrot is frequently added in cleansing diets because of its fiber and vitamin contents. It is also good for the skin which is one of the exit ways for trapped toxins inside the body.

Your cleansing program will benefit from the inclusion of potatoes in your homemade recipes as this can assist in the development of muscle mass. You will therefore lose weight by shedding of water and fats, and not by lowering your muscle mass. Consuming potatoes will also provide you with a feeling of fullness so you will not experience intense food cravings while carrying out a detox program.

Ingredients:

1 tbsp. Olive oil
4 Carrots (diced)
2 Potatoes (diced)
1 Onion (chopped)
1 inch Ginger (sliced into strips)

3 cups Water
1 tsp. Thyme

Procedure:

1. Rinse all ingredients under running water to get rid of soil, dust, and pesticides.

2. In a soup pot, sauté the onion and ginger in 1 tbsp of olive oil.

3. Add the diced carrots and potatoes, and 3 cups of water.

4. Bring to a boil.

5. Add 1 tsp. of thyme.

6. Simmer until the carrots and potatoes are soft.

7. Serve hot.

Veggie-Veggie Detox Drink

This recipe is a really potent drink as it is mainly comprised of vegetable ingredients. All the components are fresh, so you can be sure that all the essential vitamins and minerals are preserved during its creation.

Carrot is one of the main ingredients of this simple recipe as it adds nutritional value and pleasant taste to the final resulting drink. The green leafy veggies are also full of fiber which is essential in a detox program, and they carry high levels of B vitamins too.

Even in minimal portions, the onion and garlic components of this recipe also add nutritional value to the juice as these are both considered as antioxidants. The body is therefore guarded against free radicals, and proper elimination of toxic substances in the system is also supported.

Ingredient:

2 Carrots
2 Kale leaves
1 Celery stalk
1 Beet
1 Turnip
½ cup Spinach
½ cup Parsley
½ cup Cabbage
1 Onion
3 Garlic cloves

Procedure:

1. Wash all the ingredients to make sure that they are free from dirt and chemicals.

2. Put all of the produce in the juicer or blender. Make sure that you roll the leafy veggies to add density while processing.

3. Drink immediately and put any leftover portion in the refrigerator for later consumption.

Cranberry and Apple Juice

This is another simple recipe that you can easily make at home when you are on a cleansing diet. Both fruits are high in vitamin C, and they are also full of fiber which is needed for proper waste disposal.

Aside from its detoxifying properties, Cranberries can also cure urinary tract infection naturally, so it's like targeting 2 different agendas all at once.

Ingredients:

2 cups Cranberries
2 Red apples

Procedure:

1. Wash the fruits under running water as these may be contaminated with pesticides.

2. Slice the apples in chunks and remove the seeds.

3. Put both ingredients in the blender or juicer.

4. Enjoy the drink chilled or with ice.

Chapter 11: Should You Do a Body Detox?

The body will have renewed strength when you clean up the system from poisonous substances and toxic elements. As pollutants and contaminants are present in the water, air, and food products that are regularly consumed, the body is exposed to a wide variety of ailments. This makes a person prone to simple sickness like colds and flu to life-threatening diseases like cancer and heart problems. By adapting body detox programs, any toxic build-up will be eliminated from the system gradually so that the blood, tissues, and organs will remain healthy and functioning well.

You can look at a body detox procedure as a way to cleanse and nourish the body both inside and out. The process mainly involves a method to remove harmful chemicals from the system through a series of steps, while providing a healthy source of nutrients for the body as well. Toxins are therefore released through the major organs of the body (lungs, kidneys, lymph, skin, and colon).

As a detox plan mainly involves a change in one's diet, it is recommended that you consult a doctor first. Moreover, you should also consult a nutritionist or dietician so that a particular meal plan can be modified or adjusted to suit your own requirements.

Body detox can be done once to four times a year, depending on the intensity of the program and the state of one's health. While it is important to keep a well-cleansed system, it is not advisable to carry out detox procedures too frequently as it can result in nutritional deficiency.

All in all, regular body detox has been known to deliver positive results. Aside from making a person feel better by having renewed energy, it can also give the immune system a boost. As the body produces new and healthier cells, it will be more resistant to stress and diseases.

www.ingramcontent.com/pod-product-compliance
Lightning Source LLC
Chambersburg PA
CBHW070316290526
45791CB00003B/1131